DOCTORS SAID THAT I WOULD NEVER USE MY HAND AGAIN

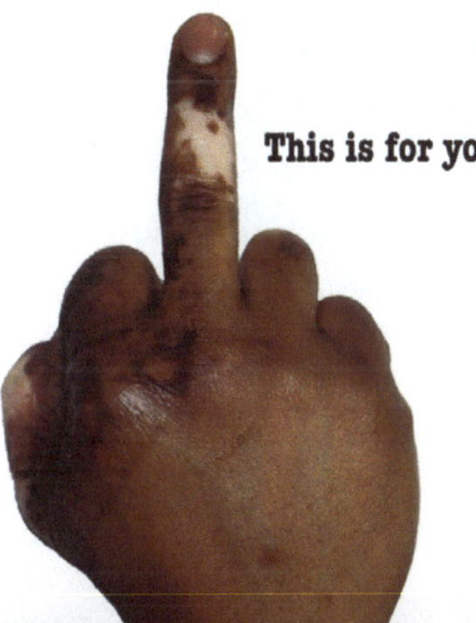

BURN HAND TREATMENT

A HOW-TO GUIDE FOR REHABILITATION, WITH REAL LIFE EXPERIENCES DIRECTLY FROM A BURN SURVIVOR

JOSH JORDAN

DISCLAIMER

The material in this book is for informational purposes only. As each individual situation is unique, you should use proper discretion, and consult with a health care practitioner, before undertaking any exercises, techniques or advice described in this book. The author expressly disclaims responsibility for any adverse effects that may result from the use of the information contained in this book.

CONTENTS

INTRO TO MY STORY

INTRO TO
MY STORY

You could call me a fitness coach, a friend, a brother and more recently a burn victim. But I do not wish for this misfortune to define me. I have been through a lot in my life and I look at my burn as just another chapter in the book of life. I have broken bones, torn muscles, been violently ill and concussed, but I do have to say that being burned is at the top of the list of pain and discomfort. If you are reading this, I am assuming that you have been burned, know someone who has been burned or are wondering about being burned, and I want you to be as prepared as possible for this experience, because I sure as hell wasn't!

I wish that I had had a first-hand report (no pun intended) about what I was about to go through, just to have a point of reference or some reassurance, so that I would not have felt so alone. Any new experience can be scary if you have unanswered questions and don't know what to expect. If this book can help even one person feel less alone in their rehabilitation journey, then I'll be happy.

The actual moment that you are being burned can be quite traumatic, but the real pain begins after the burn, when the skin starts healing. Your nervous system is constantly sending signals throughout your body to make sure everything is in order. In my case, I was missing muscle tissue, skin and cartilage, and this sent out waves of panic signals, triggering my pain sensors and that was very hard to deal with. I found that I constantly had to remind myself that I was strong enough to get through it, and that one day it would all be just a memory. Anyone can tap into this same resolve and strength; all you have to do is accept it.

Unfortunately, I had to figure out how to rehabilitate my hand on my own, as the medical system didn't provide me with much assistance. The doctors told me that they had seen burns like mine before and that my hand was a lost cause. That meant No rehab, No surgery and No help from the system. I'm lucky that I was born stubborn and refused to go along with what those doctors were trying to convince me to be fact. They might know their textbooks, but they didn't know me, and I refused to believe that my hand would just be a useless piece of meat. I still had many hands to shake, high fives to give and ladders to climb.

If you are at all like me, then you will be willing to try almost anything to get rid of the discomfort and get back to a "normal" state. If you do have this type of mentality, then life can get really expensive. I checked out so many different skin products that I quickly became a shopping channel junkie. I was always on the lookout for the next new "skin crack" so the "buy now" button quickly translated into a "fix me now" button. I had never been an impulse shopper before, but it's funny how money and bills lose all meaning when you're going through something difficult and feeling desperate to find anything that works.

After many months of experimenting and doing my own rehabilitation, I'm extremely happy and proud to be able to say that I have regained full functionality of my hand, despite all odds! Can you hear me clapping?

I spent thousands of dollars on creams, oils and special bandages. I also spent countless hours online researching anything that could give my skin more elasticity, strength and color. I dedicated so much time and energy, that it almost felt like a job.

I did all the work, so you don't have to.

I am writing this in hopes that all that work will help other people, who unfortunately, are where I was. I remember how lost I felt, and all the negative thoughts that plagued me, so once again, if this helps one person avoid any of that, then it will have all been worth it.

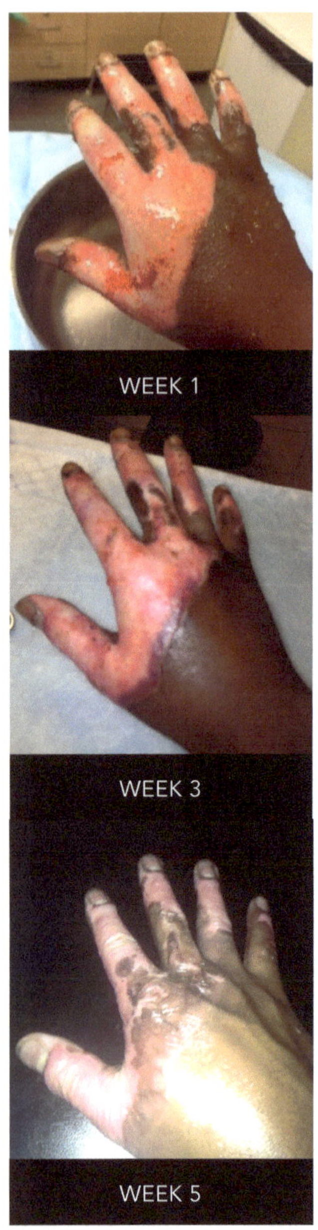

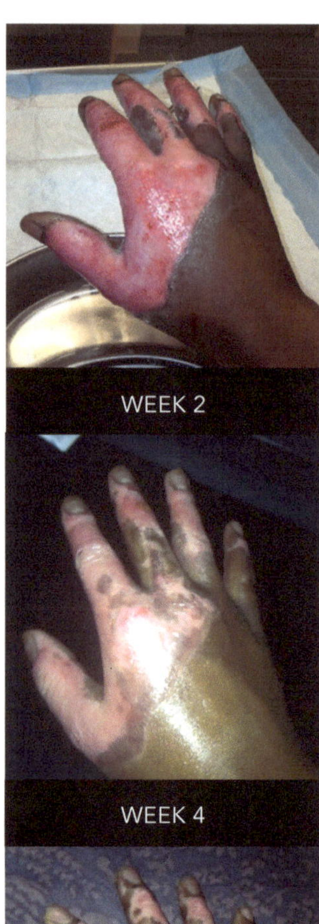

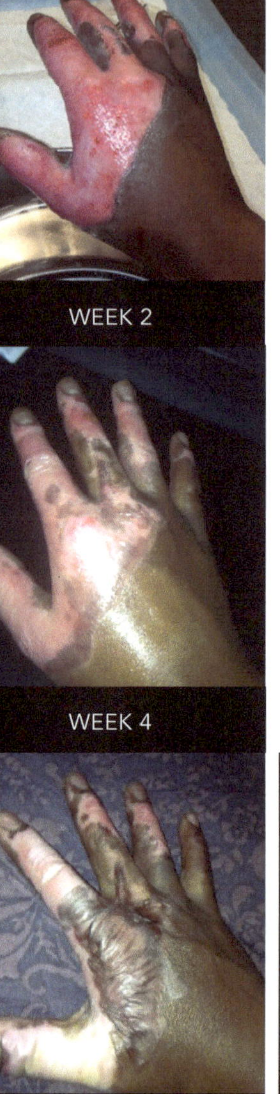

"I NEVER STOPPED BELIEVING IN ME; NEVER STOP BELIEVING IN YOU."

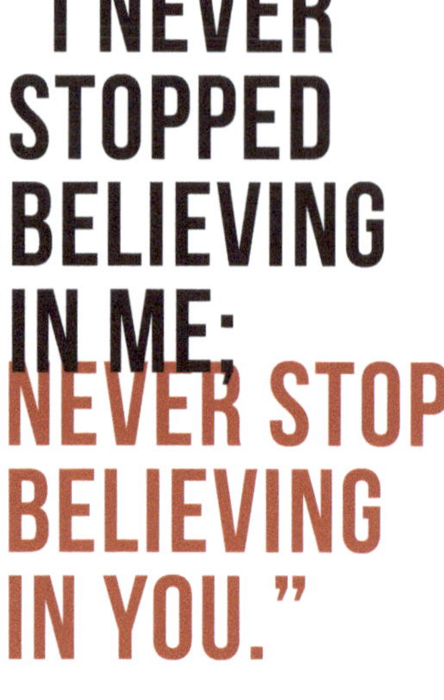

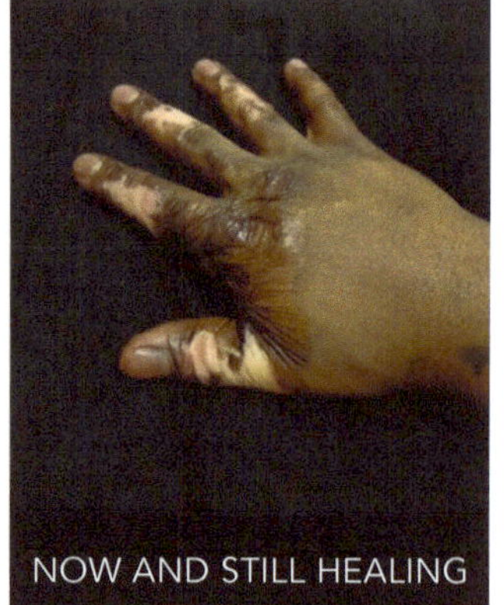

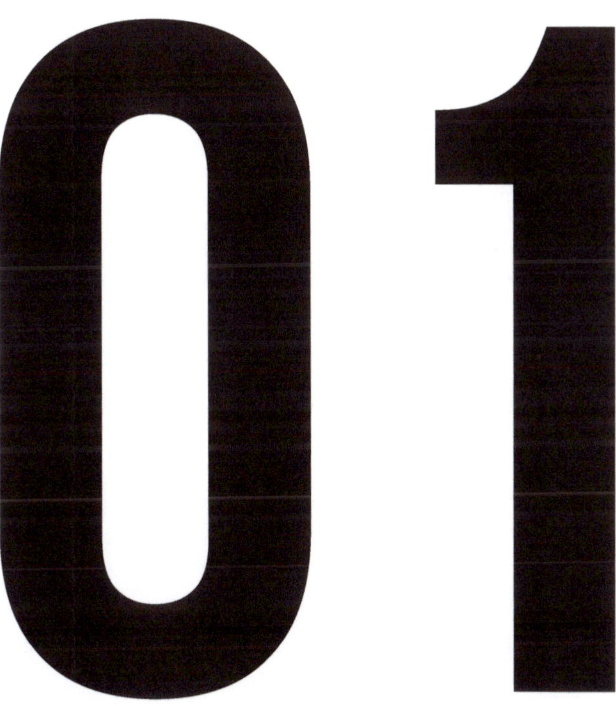

CHAPTER 1

You've been burned...
Now what?

Hi! My name is Josh Jordan and this is the story of my burn. Three years ago I was in the best shape of my life. I took care of myself, had great relationships with my friends and family and had all kinds of plans for travelling and personal projects. One day I was in my apartment enjoying a quiet day in, cooking and listening to music. I was standing in front of the stove cooking some lunch when I saw a flicker below the pan on my stove, and before I knew it there was a bon fire in front of me. Naturally, I started to panic, then went into fire fighter mode to put out the inferno that was trying to claim my apartment. There I was standing in front of this fire that could easily harm me but the first things that came to mind were losing my apartment, my shoes, my clothes and my electronics. In that first moment I wasn't thinking about myself at all. How did I become so programmed and shallow that I was more concerned with being stylish than with my own well–being. We came into this world free from possessions and that's how we will leave it, we need to focus more on ourselves rather than the things we own or can own. Wow that was an eye opener! My priorities were completely warped.

You hear all kinds of amazing things about what adrenaline can do to the body, including suppressing the pain inflicted from injuries. It's a whole other story to experience it first hand, I didn't even feel that my hand was on fire until I looked at it and saw the "Ghost Rider" blue flame outlining my right hand. My writing hand!!! The thing that concerns me the most about this situation is that as soon as I realized that my hand was on fire, all the flames went out, on the stove and on my hand at the same time. This makes me think that I was supposed to be burned for a reason (cue in sci-fi music).

My father was in a similar situation, more than a decade ago, he worked on ships and one day he was walking on deck and slipped overboard. Naturally he reached out to save himself from falling into unknown waters, but in doing so his arm met a jagged piece of metal in the hull of the ship. It ripped open his wrist and forearm and left his hand immobilized. He did nothing more than the physiotherapy that he was prescribed and still to this day he has not regained the strength in his hand. From the start he was convinced that he was a victim and wouldn't be able to overcome what had happened to him. His arteries, veins and ligaments were surgically repaired, but they might just as well not have been, since he had already accepted to live a physically challenged life. I remember reading somewhere that "the unconquered challenges of the father are passed down to the son." At the time I had no clue what that meant for me but now, it is a lot clearer. I believe that my experience in comparison to his, teaches the lesson that what you choose to believe truly molds your reality.

Let me paint you a picture. I had just gotten burned, I was sitting down clutching my wrist with sweat dripping from every part of my body, as the heat from the fire was slowly dissipating. I looked down in disbelief to see my hand looking like a stiff, old, frayed piece of leather and once again I went into panic mode. All the negative thoughts started to flood in the gates.

"This can't be my hand!"

"I must be dreaming!"

"How could this have happened to me?!"

I started frantically searching the Internet for ways to dull the burning sensation I was feeling. This only made things worse, as I was not able to find anything to reassure me and give me that "everything will be okay" feeling.

My first instinct was to stuff my hand in the freezer to cool down but I was met with a steak (that I had always meant to cook) which was heavily freezer burned. The fire already burned my hand and I wasn't going to let ice get in on the action too! My gut was right because I later spoke with a nurse friend of mine, Amelie, and she told me that it was good that I hadn't added ice. She explained to me that the skin was already damaged from the burn and that exposure to cold would have made my skin prone to frost bite. The cold of the ice would have also slowed down the blood flow and prolonged the healing process. That steak was just another reminder that everything happens for a reason.

While I was waiting for my lift to the hospital I kept scouring the Internet for quick pain remedies. I came across an article by George Krucik MD, who provides consulting for Healthline.com.

He said that using cool to room temperature water would alleviate some of the burning sensation. This was not the haymaker that I was hoping for, but it was better than nothing. I soaked an old t-shirt (nothing with loose or protruding fibers that could stick to the wound) in lukewarm water and wrapped my hand in it. I then found a cooler and filled it with warm water and dunked my wrapped hand into that and made my way to the hospital.

Here I was walking into the packed emergency room with my hand in a cooler and the expressions of pain and anger written all over my face. I felt like I was the star of an action film and this was my anticlimax. They must have predicted that the madman was about to be unleashed because I didn't even have to wait two minutes before two surgeons showed up. That has to be some kind of record! The only thing on my mind at the time was the pain and getting rid of it, so I was feeling very pro-drugs.

I couldn't believe it, but the surgeon said that the pain couldn't be that bad and that I could wait until he was done the assessment before giving me pain pills. I almost felt like lighting his hand on fire, just to see if he would still feel the same way. I was both surprised and disappointed at this type of response, and I knew, this wasn't anything minor. After they cut the dead skin from my hand I realized that the pain I had been feeling was only the little brother, and the mean big brother had just stepped in. The air touching my open wound felt like Lingchi, the ancient torture of 1000 cuts. Let's just say that I got my pain treatment much sooner than after the assessment.

The doctors advised me that I had third degree burns and that the damage done was irreversible. I was told that I would not get any of my pigmentation back and as a black man that meant my scarring would be substantial, and very obvious. Even more shocking, was when they said that I would not regain the use of my hand.

I don't know how the medical system got so messed up. I thought they were meant to patch you up and send you home feeling better; not crush all of your hopes and dreams and then kick you to the curb.

That sent me into a depression. I started thinking about where I would go next with my life.

"Who would want someone with one working hand?"

"How will I drive?"

"How will I work out, climb, or even pick myself up if I fall?"

"Will I need to be assisted the rest of my life?"

Looking back now I feel a bit silly having thought like that but we humans tend to jump to the worst conclusions, and taking the word of an "expert" seemed like my only option at the time. Those doctors might have been experts in their theories, but none of them were experts on me.

02

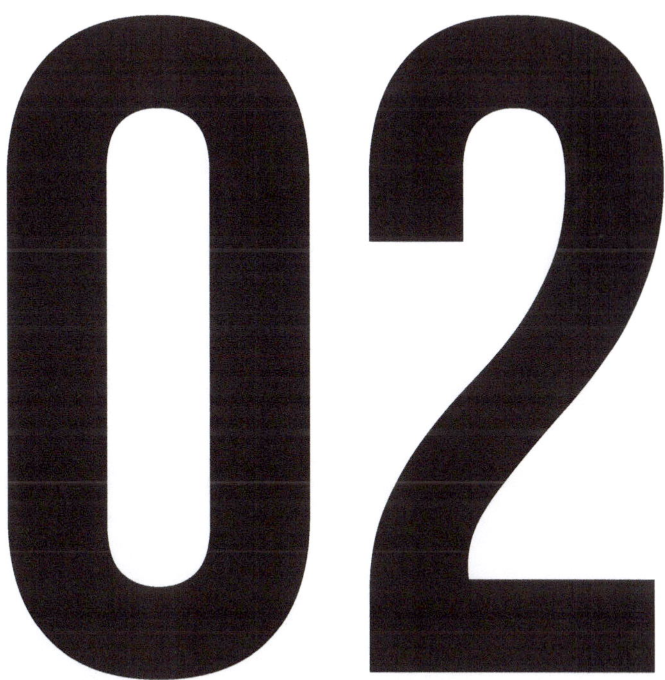

CHAPTER 2

What to expect from
the healing process

DAY 2 -

After the initial hospital visit I had to start getting my bandages changed. I didn't know at the time that the process was going to be so difficult, but the next five weeks were going to be my personal little hell. Every day the scars begin to form and harden only to be ripped open again when the bandages were removed and replaced with new ones. If you have already gone through this experience, then you know exactly what I mean, and if you haven't, my goal here isn't to scare, but to prepare you.

In the beginning I wasn't able to change my own bandages so I had to go to the CLSC, which is a governed local community service center that provides nurses and health services in Quebec, Canada (you more than likely have a similar service in your area). I constantly had to buy packages of medicated bandages and Flamazine cream (over the counter burn ointment). The box of bandages came four in a pack (each about 4 inches x 6 inches) and the cream was in 20g tubes. The bandages were about $15-$20 a box depending on the pharmacy, and the cream was around $8 a tube. The cream was covered by my insurance but the bandages… Surprise, surprise they were not. I needed both every day and the box of bandages would only be good for two usages, if I was lucky, and the cream would last about five or six usages. Let's just say that the fire burned my hand and a hole through my wallet.

I had burns on my whole hand, so the inside and outside and each finger needed to be covered separately, so it kind of looked like a catcher's mitt. It was a tedious process; let me break it down for you:

1. Removal of bandages

2. Cleansing of the wounds with water and saline solution

3. Cutting away all dead skin

4. Application of Flamazine cream to the wounds

5. Application of bandages over the cream

6. Wrapping of the whole hand in gauze (thank the lord this was provided free)

OH AND DID I MENTION THAT THIS WAS EVERYDAY!?

I remember dreading going in to the clinic because often times it wouldn't be the same nurse. Would I get a sweet gentle nurse, or would I get a "bandage you up and get the f*ck out" kind? In a burned state any kind of touch is going to be painful so you need to take that extra care to not cause further damage. I had to ban two nurses from my file, not so much for my well-being, but for theirs. A few of the survivors I keep in contact with, also had similar experiences. I guess that's to be expected when dealing with people providing service, sometimes it's just a job and they forget that the goal is to help. That being said I really do hope that you have the best experience with that as possible.

Around three and half weeks in I couldn't deal with going to the clinic anymore, so I decided to tough it out on my own and put the bandages on myself for the next couple of weeks. I had seen enough poor attempts by nurses to know exactly what not to do, so I was feeling pretty confident. By this time I had gotten to know the staff and they supplied me with everything. They pulled out bandages, gauze, sterilized scissors and tweezers, but I still had to buy my own cream. This is probably the only time in my life that I enjoyed being pitied because it saved me money and time.

I became a pro at my bandages after only a few days and only had to go to the clinic once a week just to get more supplies. I salvaged hours of my time not having to go there daily.
If you get to a point where you are doing it yourself, make sure that you use a designated clean and sterilized area. The very last thing that you want to do is catch an infection. Don't reuse tools unless they are sterilized as this isn't the time to be lazy or cheap. Your health needs to be a priority. An infection would really set you back in the healing department and could cause even further damage to your already fragile skin. Infections can break down the skin, while you are trying to do the exact opposite, regenerate it.

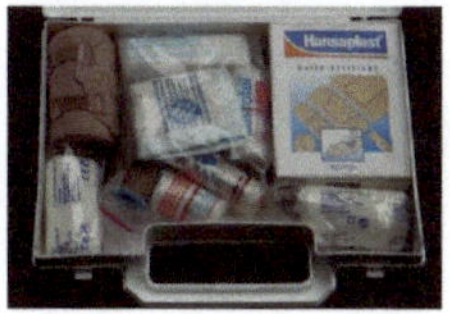

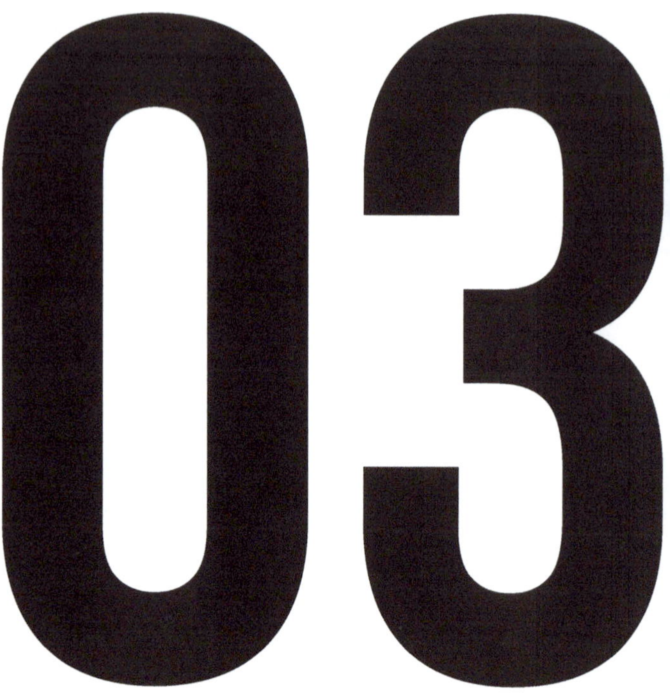

03

TAKE CONTROL OF
YOUR SELF ESTEEM

There's nothing like a traumatic experience that swoops in to change your outlook on life. It really is a telltale moment that defines what kind of person you are going to be. I could have decided to listen to the doctor's predictions and let my hand become useless. This was only if I wanted to believe that my life was going to control me, instead of me controlling my life.

START SHARING YOUR STORY because you never know how your story can help someone else. Doing this can provide a win-win outcome because not only could you help others, but the more you tell your story, the more at peace you will feel about your situation. The more at peace you are with your situation, the better you will feel about it. It will quickly become just a story about an event in your life and it will lose its power over you.

I'm not saying that this is easy, because at the beginning it will be difficult reliving what happened over and over again. I am naturally a private person, I had difficulty with sharing but over time it got easier and allowed me to become more open about life and myself in general.

At the very beginning people would see my hand and stare, some would even muster up the courage to ask me what happened. My first reactions were to just say that I got burned and leave it at that. I thought that avoidance would be the best medicine, but I quickly found out that I was wrong.

One day I was getting my car washed and I saw the car wash owner's eyes darting back and forth from my hand. I figured I would be there a while, so I could give my usual quick answer and stand there awkwardly for the rest of my wait or I could just share my story with him. I chose to tell him and I got an unexpected response. He started telling me about his burn story; when he was a child he was in a house fire and got badly burned. He took off his shirt, right there in the garage and he had burn scars down his neck, back and chest. It didn't seem to faze him at all! I had to ask how he had gotten through it, especially as a child, since children can be so cruel. He told me a story that his grandmother told him, which helped him through the acceptance of his scars. She told him that everyone would have to have their sins burned out of them, before going to heaven. Since he had already been burned, he would end up going straight there. I am not much of a religious person, but this story still gave me quite a bit of satisfaction. I felt like I was part of an exclusive club that was already green lit for the VIP section, and it gave me comfort.

"SOMETIMES YOU CAN'T GET SOMEONE ELSE'S TRUTH UNLESS YOU OFFER UP YOUR OWN."

WEAR YOUR SCARS
LIKE A BADGE,

surviving something as life threatening as fire is a huge triumph. I was only able to realize this once I took myself out of the equation, because you can't see the picture when you are in the frame. Initially, when you are so close to a situation, you aren't able to see the bright side. Of course it was bad that I got burned, but it could have been much worse. In my small apartment, a fire like that could have quickly gotten out of control and given me more burns, or even have taken my life. I am counting every minute, hour and day as a blessing and my scars are a constant reminder of that.

You have to think that as long as you have visible scars, there will be someone with questions. You'd be amazed at the number of people who will actually feel uncomfortable because they want to know, but don't want to ask. I often catch the eye movements of people, I can tell want to ask, but don't have the courage. If it is someone significant in my life, and I catch them looking, I will normally say something right away. At the beginning I was quite shy about the state of my hand and I found that feeding their curiosity shifted the balance of awkwardness. After hearing the story they would be more focused on the "what if it happened to them?" scenario and most vocalize that I am strong for getting through it. I was also very worried about dating again because I was feeling very self-conscious. I was doing the online dating thing for a while and I won't lie, not everyone is very accepting. But that was their loss because I'm amazing!!! I soon learned that there are bigger issues when dating complete strangers than just some scars. At the end of the day, you need to get out of your own head and just put yourself out there.

Remember, everyone has scars, the only difference is yours are visible to the naked eye.

"DON'T BE ASHAMED BECAUSE YOU WEAR YOUR STRUGGLE ON YOUR SKIN."

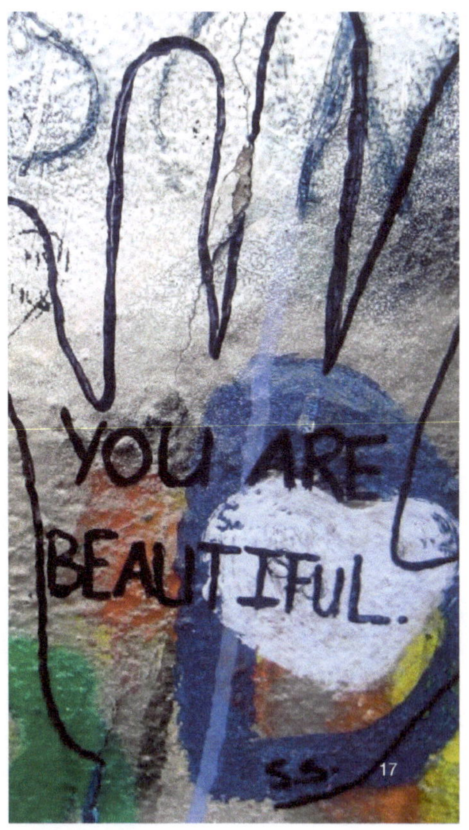

CREATE AN ANCHOR
FOR YOUR SCARS

in order to eliminate the powers they have over you and for you to gain power over your mind. First off, an anchor more specifically a mental anchor is a link in your mind that connects one thing to another. For example, when you hear the popular jingle "ba da, da da da, I'm loving it" you automatically think of McDonalds (you probably even just sang it in your head). So what you need to do is create a similar link for your scars. You want to associate your scars with a good feeling of strength and power, to override the negative feelings.

1. Sit down and write out in as much detail as you can, all the times you can remember when you felt uplifted, accomplished and proud of yourself.

2. When you're done, read them to yourself and pick the two that you can see the clearest in your mind's eye.

3. These two scenarios are now going to represent the new emotions that you are going to feel about your scars.

4. Now stare at your scars until you feel like you can still see them when you close your eyes.

5. Once your eyes are closed and you are visualizing your scars, now start thinking about your first inspiring scenario. Try and see it like a movie in your head. Remember how you felt, letting all the good and free emotions flow through your body. Continue until your thoughts begin to fade.

6. Now repeat steps 4 and 5 with your second inspiring scenario.

7. Repeat this every day until you feel your mind shift and you start thinking differently about your scars.

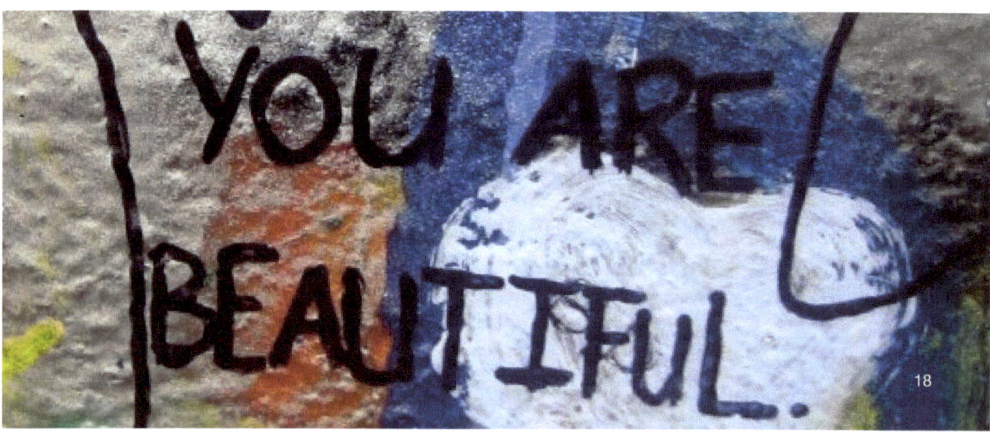

SHIFT YOUR FOCUS

and pay attention to the positive side of your story. It's a natural instinct to remain focused on the bad side of things because from the beginning of human life it has been a life-saving instinct. Way back before Facebook, shopping malls and fast cars, we used to live in caves among wild animals. Back then it could have saved your life to automatically think that the rustling in a bush was a predator to stay clear of. Back then many things could have been seen as a threat and the "better safe than sorry" response would kick in. We now live in a much safer environment, where going out to grab food isn't a life or death experience (well, in my environment anyways). I suppose if you live in a war torn environment your focus might be different.

The core 'fight or flight' instinct of the human brain hasn't evolved as quickly as the world around us. So while thinking cynically could have saved our ancestors' lives, we now apply this type of thinking to every aspect of our lives. We have adopted this cynical bias and in this day and age it hurts us more than being beneficial to us. It actually takes longer to appreciate positivity than negativity. Negative thinking is on autopilot and has an almost instant effect, in comparison to positive thinking, that takes about five seconds to really resonate with us. Have you ever been in an argument with someone and no matter what they say, you just want to tell them that they are wrong? Only later on, after you have had time to think about it, you realize you could have handled the situation better? This comes from the negative bias, and the ego, but that's a whole different topic in itself.

Basically what I want you to take away from this is to take your time and analyze situations before you react. There is almost always more than one way to think about, or to approach a situation. If you feel like you have to absolutely give the negativity some thought, then think of how bad it could have been. You could've been burned to death, but you are alive and have a chance at doing something with your life.

"DON'T CRY WHEN THE CANVAS DOESN'T TURN OUT HOW YOU EXPECTED. CRY WHEN THERE IS NO CANVAS LEFT."

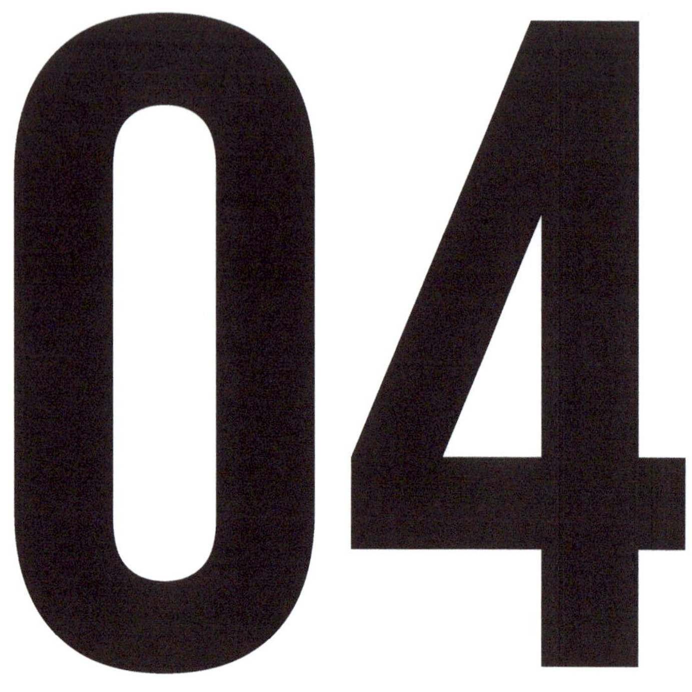

04

CHAPTER 4

D.I.Y rehab

D.I.Y REHAB

Yes! Yes I did, I had to rehab my hand on my own. Looking back, I'm actually happy that it turned out this way because this process has made me stronger. If I had been assigned a physiotherapist that I would have seen regularly, then I would have mentally assigned the responsibility of having rehabilitated my hand to someone else. Nobody knows your limits and thresholds better than you, and nobody will have your best interests in mind better than you. That being said, I'm not saying to fire your physiotherapist. I would actually suggest taking full advantage of all the help that you can get. Just remember that at the end of the day, getting your hand back into fighting shape is your battle and an hour or two here and there with physio isn't going to work wonders. For this exact reason, I will be sharing with you the exercises that you can do on your own to increase your mobility over time.

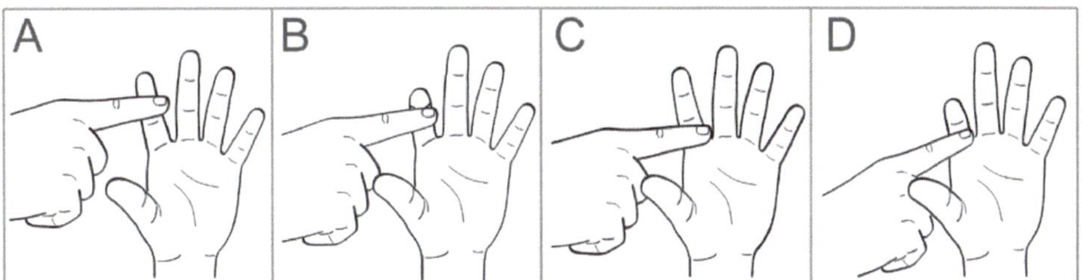

Use your opposite hand to apply pressure below each joint of the finger to isolate the joint and bend your finger as much as you can and hold for 5 seconds. Repeat this with each finger.

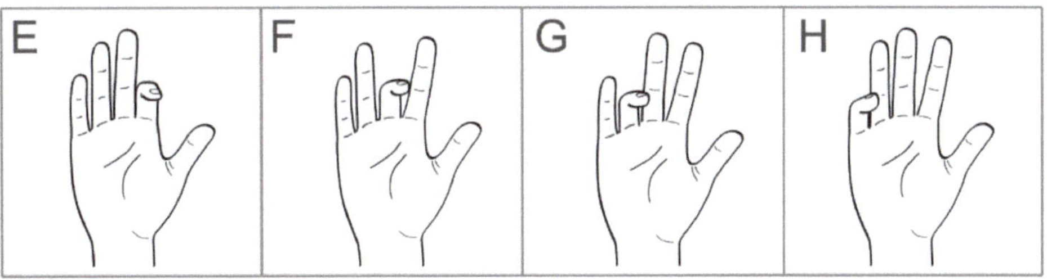

Bend your finger as much as you can and hold for 5 seconds. Repeat with each finger.

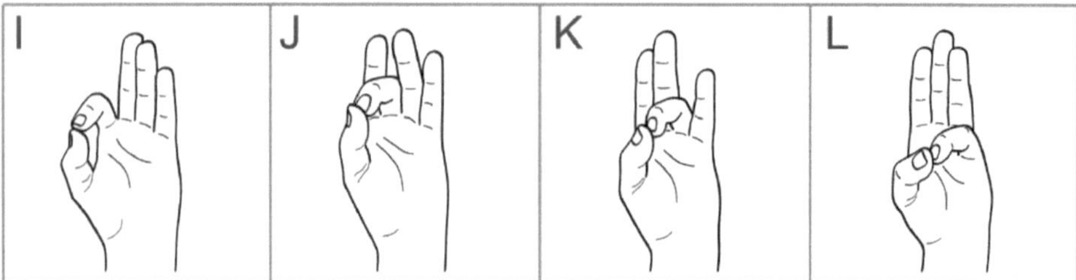

Touch the tip of your thumb to the tip of each finger (or as close as you can get it)
and hold for 5 seconds.

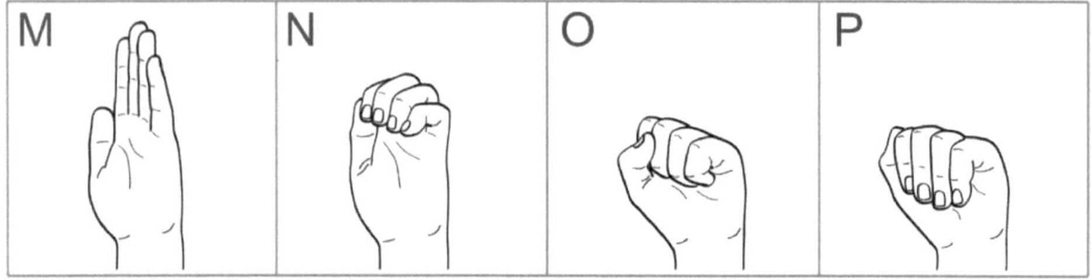

Slowly try to make a fist (or as much of a fist as you can) and hold for 5 seconds. Then
touch the tips of your fingers to the bottom of your palm and hold for 5 seconds.

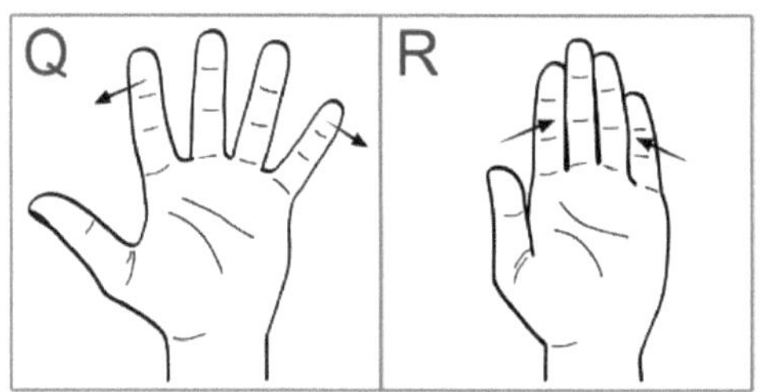

Spread your fingers as far apart as possible and hold for 5 seconds and
then bring them back together.

SET YOURSELF A 20 MINUTE TIMER AND DO AS MANY OF THESE EXERCISES AS
YOU CAN IN 20 MINUTES AT LEAST TWICE A DAY.

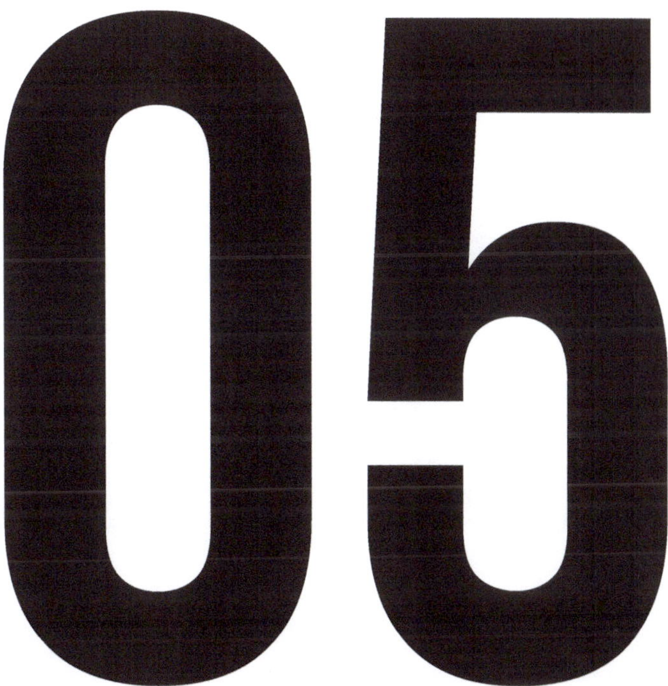

05

CHAPTER 5

Revisit your diet
rejuvenate your skin

REVISIT YOUR DIET
REJUVENATE YOUR SKIN

It is usually when you hit bottom that you really take a look at your life choices and try to make a serious change. For so many years I have been a person that worked out, so I always thought that I was doing enough to be healthy. It was only after being hospitalized for being nutrient deficient that I really understood the importance of getting the right nutrients. Everything does happen for a reason and most times the reason is nowhere in sight when the unexpected happens. Experiences are meant to make you stronger, mentally or physically so that you are better prepared to handle future events. Unknowingly the knowledge that I got when I was sick in the hospital prepared me for battling my burns. I've always been amazed by the human body, and people who are constantly showing us that our limits can be pushed. It goes to show that we as a human race have not even scratched the surface of our own possibilities. With the right tools and direction we can achieve just about anything.

Your skin is constantly shedding and regenerating but your body needs the right nutrients to be able to produce smooth skin with elasticity. Luckily you can get all the right nutrients just by eating the right things. There are many natural foods that can assist you in your healthy skin goal but I would like to share the ones that helped me get to where I am today.

• Spinach and Kale – Spinach and kale are two leafy green veggies that are packed full of vitamins that help repair and rejuvenate the skin. I put them in my daily green smoothies and they became a big part of how I regrew my skin.

• Potassium is a key element in these leafy greens and is an electrolyte that conducts energy in the body. It's a building block for the proper functioning of cells and muscles, so yes I would say it's quite important for your skin's regrowth and your body as a whole. I had an experience several years ago of being hospitalized, almost incoherent because I was potassium deficient, this is just an example of learning from your experiences.

• Iron is responsible for moving around oxygen in your red blood cells, to get from your lungs and heart to the rest of your body. If your body isn't getting enough oxygen then it definitely won't be able to heal itself.

• Vitamin K helps reduce dry, itchy skin. These are two symptoms that were extremely annoying and drove me crazy during the healing process. My skin was so sensitive that I couldn't scratch so I had to pat my hand all the time and it looked like I was disciplining myself. Putting cream on the skin can only go so far for hydrating when your skin can't hold moisture. Dry skin can make mobility very painful; the skin is tight and tough to move. This makes trying to rehabilitate very hard, because it is difficult to move when your body is fighting against you. The dryness and itching got a lot better after I started drinking my green smoothies. I drank them every day and started seeing a very noticeable change at the three week mark of ingesting them. Very similar to working out, it takes about three weeks for your body to recognize the new habit.

With all this smoothie talk, I might as well share the recipe, so here it is:

SMOOTHIE RECIPE:

For a green smoothie to be a green smoothie and get all the benefits you need to follow the ratio 4:2. You have to have 4 greens for every 2 fruits. You can find the ingredients to my "Go To" green smoothie here:

1 handful of de-stemmed spinach

1 handful of kale

1/2 a cucumber chopped up

1 head of broccoli

1 grapefruit skinned and sliced

1 green apple chopped up

1 lime skinned and sliced

1 cup of water

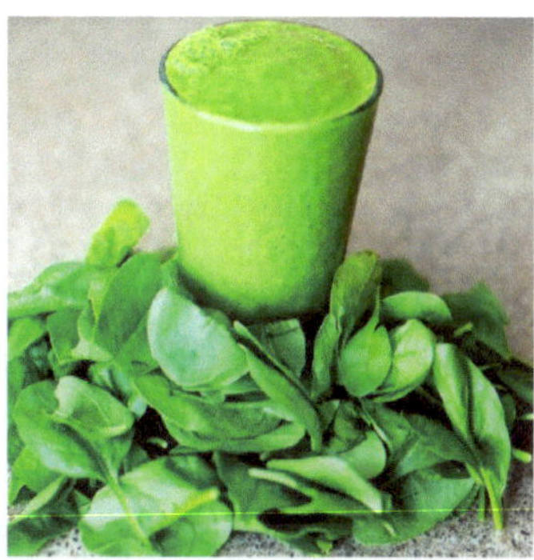

This mix will give you a very green taste, but you can substitute the green apple or grapefruit for a banana if you prefer a sweeter taste. Now for blending these together, there is an order you have to follow so that it ends up smooth instead of clumpy. Pour in about a cup of water; leafy greens next, one at a time until each is well blended then you add everything else one at a time. It should end up being pretty smooth, but feel free to add more water to make it smoother if needed. The fibers from all the greens will act like a toothbrush to clean out your insides. If you don't tend to be very regular, you will be shortly!

PINEAPPLES WATER

Pineapples not only taste great, they're good for you too. They have an active ingredient called bromelain that does all kinds of wonderful things for your body but I'll be focusing on one.

· It is a natural anti-inflammatory, so that means it gets rid of puffiness, redness and stiffness in skin. I always loved pineapple, but I only found out about this after a jaw surgery I had around 11 years ago from a football injury. My face was so swollen that it made it hard to speak, and that was more than annoying and it helped me get rid of the swelling. I was drinking pure pineapple juice every day and when that started to get pricey, I started taking bromelain pills. My skin got a lot less puffy and tight and in just a week or two there was a very noticeable change. When something works you keep doing it, so I did the same thing when my hand was inflamed and it helped get my fingers moving quicker. Inflammation can really debilitate your mobility and hinder you on your road to rehab success, so getting rid of inflammation is a very important step in the process.

Water - believe it or not but water is going to be an instrumental tool in your quest for healthier skin. It's common knowledge that 70% of our bodies are made up of water, but a lot of us still do not get enough water in our diet. Think of what happens when a body of water like a pond doesn't get any circulating water? It starts to get stagnant and bacteria and fungus start to form. Am I right, or am I right? With this in common, we have to keep the water in our body moving. Our cells are constantly regenerating and getting rid of waste, and our bodies need water to be able to circulate nutrients and produce cells. You need to help your body out and give it a means to keep the cycle going. We do not want to give any bacteria the chance to take shelter and build a family inside us. Think of yourself like a body of water. If the waters don't flow then it turns into a swamp. Keep the flow going so that the line keeps moving and there is no time to stop and latch on. In with the good and out with the bad. It is said that the human body should have around three-four liters (just under a gallon) of water a day. That does sound like a lot, but there is also water in a lot of the things that we eat, so that is also taken into account. What I did is I went and picked up a one liter water bottle and I kept filling it up throughout the day. How you know that you are on the right track is when your urine is almost clear.

"KEEP THE RIVERS OF YOUR BODY FLOWING TO KEEP YOUR BODILY FUNCTIONS GOING."

JUNK FOOD

Limit junk food – Yes life is all about balance, but I did say limit not cut out, because that would just be crazy! There are way too many delicious things in this world that aren't the healthiest for you, but all the same, everything should be in moderation. The problem with junk food is that they are usually just empty or unhealthy calories. Your body needs nutrients, and every time that you eat you are giving your body a chance to replenish. If you aren't giving your body those nutrients then you are just cheating yourself of a healthy life.

SPIRULINA

Spirulina – This is a blue algae (seaweed) that is a super food, we could potentially live off of it, and it is very healthy, although I wouldn't suggest it as it's not the tastiest food. Spirulina is completely plant based and apparently has been around for millions of years before humans were on earth. It is mostly a protein, but also has carbohydrates, fat and a whole bunch of vitamins and minerals such as:

Vitamin A

Vitamin B-2 (riboflavin)

Vitamin B-3 (niacin)

Vitamin B-6

Vitamin C

Vitamin E

Vitamin K

Calcium

Potassium

Iron

Magnesium

Zinc

What I usually do is make a tea out of it. It comes in powder form and I put a teaspoon of it in a cup and add brown sugar (for taste) and top it off with hot water.

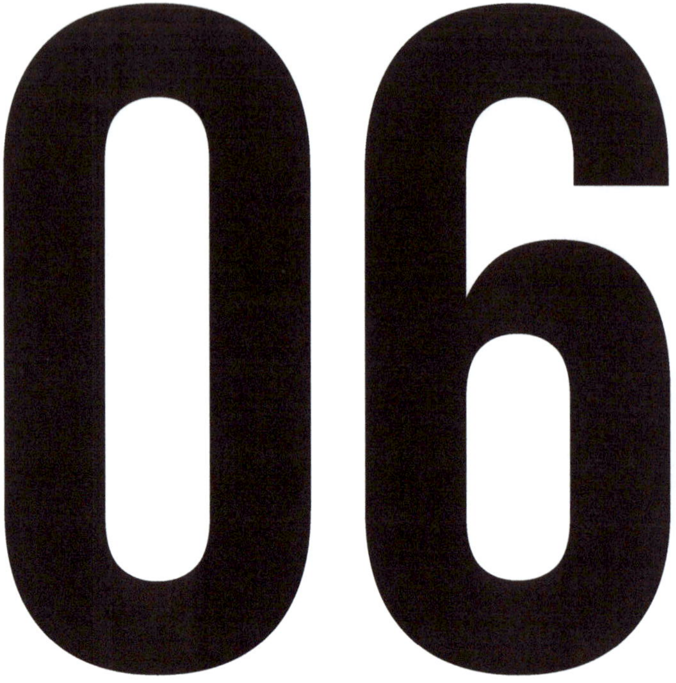

06

KEEP
HYDRATED

Massage with coconut oil- Massaging your skin will increase your circulation, reduce inflammation and get rid of dead cells. Massaging will also get rid of the buildup of stress in your hand and make it easier for you to move. The coconut oil is really hydrating and will provide you with the added moisture that your skin needs. It may be painful for you because it was for me, but you have to commit to doing it if you want to make sure that you get your hand back in functioning shape, I would massage my hand twice a day, in the morning and evening. Massage! Massage! Massage! You can do it!

Silicone disposable gloves – In the first few months after my skin formed back on my hand, my skin was incapable of keeping moisture. I had to constantly reapply creams and oils throughout the day. If I forgot, I'd quickly get a swift reminder in the form of sharp pain when I tried to move my cracked, dry skin. It was a little like having chapped lips in the winter when they would dry out and split, but increase the intensity by five… thousand!

I had to figure out a more efficient way to rehydrate my skin and I remembered what I do to keep my feet soft and smooth. I'm someone that is constantly on his feet with working out, always taking stairs and busting out a two-step whenever I can. Being active can take a toll on your feet and make them dry and callused so it is very important to take good care of them. Actually, just take good care of yourself as a whole.

Before I go to bed, I cream my feet and throw on some socks. When I wake up my feet have absorbed most of the cream and they feel much smoother. So I applied this same regimen to my hand. I made a mixture of a few natural ingredients that help rehydrate and rejuvenate skin (you can find them below).

Natural Shea butter
Tamanu oil
Natural cocoa butter
Vitamin E

REHYDRATING CREAM RECIPE

What you will need:

A small to mid-size pot
A short mason jar that will fit in the pot
3 tablespoons natural Shea butter
8-10 drops Tamanu oil
3 tablespoons natural cocoa butter
1 tablespoon vitamin E
Box of silicone disposable gloves

1. Put the pot on the stove on medium heat.

2. Pour in water up to a quarter of the pot's depth.

3. Place the mason jar in the water, in the middle of the pot.

4. Add in the Shea butter, cocoa butter, then the Tamanu oil and vitamin E.

5. Stir until mixed together, it should still have a creamy thick consistency, if it ends up too watery then add more Shea or cocoa butter.

6. Remove from heat and let cool.

For bigger batches just multiply the ingredients by two, three or four to your liking.

Congratulations! You are now a step closer to rehydrating your skin. I recommend doing this before you go to sleep. Take the cream and rub it all over your hand, put enough so that it is visible. Now take one of the silicone disposable gloves and slowly slip your hand into it making sure you don't rub off the cream. Now go to sleep!

When you wake up, your hand will be fairly wrinkly looking, as if you were in a pool for a long time. Take off the glove, (most of the cream should be absorbed) and let your hand air out. Continue to do this every night until you start to regain the ability to hold moisture.

You can use this recipe as an all day cream but due to the strong smell of the Tamanu oil it might not be too pleasant. You can make two batches, 1 for daytime minus the Tamanu, and another for the night with the Tamanu included.

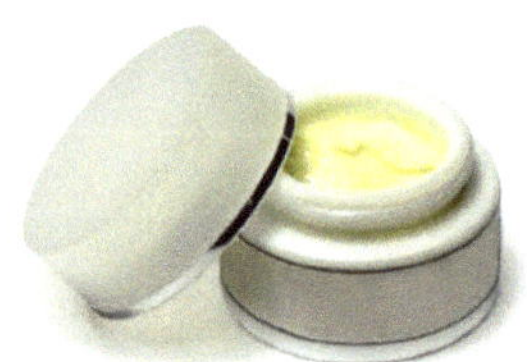

07

MIRACLE PRODUCTS

Here is a list of miracle products and my preferred brands that will help you on your road to recovery. Again, I've done all the work so that you don't have to. I've also included the clickable links so that you can get straight to the products that I used.

Spirulina http://amzn.to/28NI70f

Silicone gel sheets http://amzn.to/28Om8Jb

Tamanu oil http://amzn.to/28P2wmx

Cocoa butter http://amzn.to/28NIU1a

Shea butter http://amzn.to/28OwSVu

Bromelain pills http://amzn.to/28NIZ4Q

Jojoba oil http://amzn.to/28OwLcG

Coconut oil http://amzn.to/28P3wa6

"BELIEVE IN YOURSELF"

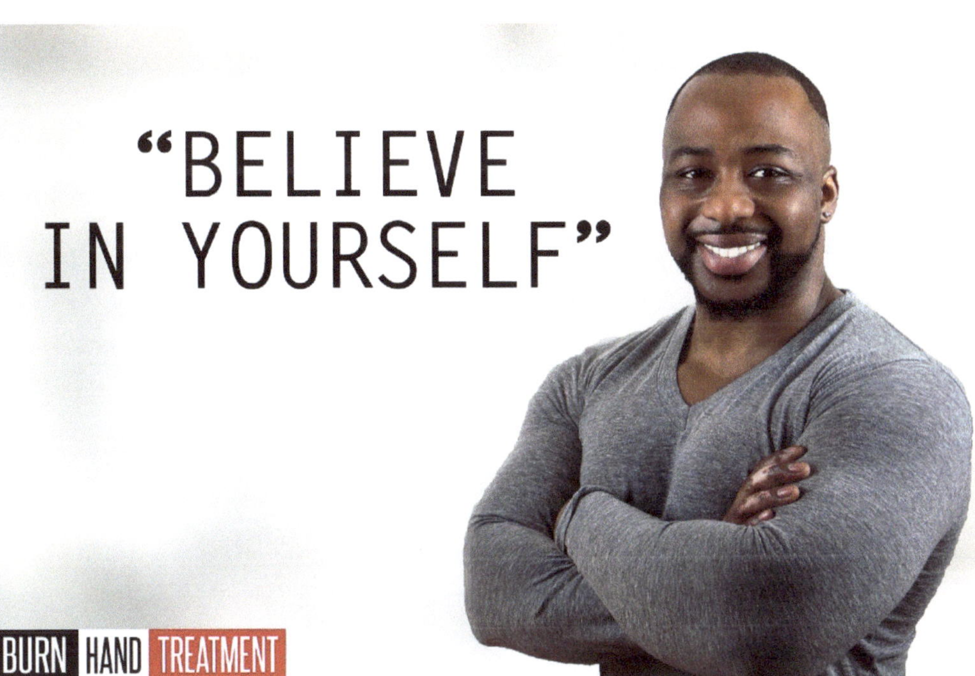

BURN HAND TREATMENT

WHAT I'VE LEARNED

To give you an update on how I am doing now, I'm doing great! My hand is stronger than it has ever been and the amazing thing is that my hand is still healing. I see new pigmentation every couple of months and I have become so accustomed to my scars that at times, I even forget that they are there. My shyness, self-consciousness and fear, are all gone. I have learned a lot about life and more importantly, about myself throughout this process. I have to admit that when I burned my hand I felt like my life was over, but to my surprise, it was the complete opposite. It was the beginning of a new chapter!

I had been working for a bank, constantly chasing the next promotion as if it was going to deliver me to the gates of happiness. The higher I got, the more I witnessed the lack of care for people and this wasn't a path that I wanted to continue on. My burn experience has given me a lot more compassion, strength and clarity. I quickly realized that there is much more to life than just working and partying. It's about the people that you have close to your heart. It's about loving yourself and others and learning from your experiences. I also learned a lot about forgiveness because I was very bitter towards the doctors that I dealt with at first. I tried to put myself in their shoes; maybe they didn't know any better; maybe it was just a job for them or maybe they were never shown compassion so they didn't know how to give it. After everything that has happened to me in my life, all I can feel is grateful because it could have been much worse and I would like to share this feeling of gratitude around.

THANK YOU, THANK YOU!

"LOVE YOURSELF EVERY DAY AND REMEMBERTO KEEP GIVING YOURSELF ANOTHER CHANCE."

I want to thank my brother Adrien for being there for me from the beginning and dropping everything to take me to the hospital, love you bruh!

I want to thank my mother Janice for taking care of me through my healing process, and doing my final edit, love you mom!

Thank you Gina for editing this book and giving your much-appreciated advice.

Thank you to my best friend Steven for always reminding me that I'm amazing, love you bruh!

Thank you Nalie for pushing me to put myself out there and also editing this book, I love you.

Thank you Justin for being my cameraman.

I also want to thank YOU for taking the time to read this book. I hope that it was able to help you.

DO'S AND DON'TS

DO

- Take responsibility for your own rehabilitation
- Exercise every day
- Keep your burn clean
- Share your story with others
- Massage your scars
- Drink three-four liters of water a day
- Moisturize your skin at least twice a day every day
- Eat healthy meals
- Take vitamins
- Get back to your regular life activities A.S.A.P
- See your scars as a Badge of Accomplishment
- Use lukewarm water to sooth burns

DON'T

- Put ice on your burn
- Reuse unsterilized tools (bandages, scissors, tweezers)
- Believe what others say about your own capabilities
- Let your burns define you
- Hide from the world

TREATMENT CALENDAR

Week 1	Week 2	Week 3	Week 4	Week 5	Week 6
• Buy products for your recovery (bandages, creams etc.) • Learn how to bandage your burn	• Start looking at ways to improve your diet to aid the healing process	• Start shifting yourself esteem	• Begin hand exercises	• Start bandaging your burn yourself	• Start hydrating your skin

SHOPPING LIST

Bandages	Bromelain pills
Spirulina	Coconut oil
Silicone gel sheets	Antiseptic cream
	Jojoba oil
Tamanu oil	Vitamin E
Cocoa butter	Disposable silicone
Shea butter	gloves